Welcome to the rest of your life.

I have created 100 workouts that can be completed in 20 minutes or less with zero gym equipment at home or on the road!

The workouts are in sequential order and are ready to start in the order set! I have even included optional rest days if using this program as a sole routine. The workouts will focus on legs, cardio, and lower/upper body strength. This program is meant to act as a functional, simple, and easy workout routine to follow. It will start you off in the right direction on your fitness journey or will give something new to confuse your muscles for the established fitness professional.

Start the rest of your life with quick, easy, at home workouts that can change your body and mind for the better.

I have been working out in 20 minutes or less for over 10 years now through my time in the Military, Diplomatic Security, and as a stay at home dad trying to save time. I have also been certified as a personal trainer from an accredited school and as a level one trainer by a famous cross training program in the past.

I am dedicated to serving the public and helping others achieve their physical or mental goals. I want to change the world, one workout or motivational quote at a time. I believe that fitness is one of the key components to living a great life.

Often, I was stranded in isolated areas with minimal gym equipment. These circumstances pushed me to create a routine that could be implemented anywhere in the world. These workouts and this standard kept me in top physical condition, capable of passing any Federal Government Physical Fitness Test. It all started with these simple workouts!

Running will become easier, fitness will become fun, and life will be better when you start a healthy workout routine.

Try these workouts and see if your fitness changes. If it does, step it up and add weight, more reps, and longer exercises. If you can't do the repetitions in the workouts or make the time limits, do as many reps as possible until failure before you move on to the next exercise.

<u>Waiver of Liability</u>

<u>Workout 1</u>:

3 Rounds For Time:

10 Air Squats (Squat to Bench or chair to scale)
20 Push-Ups (Knee Push-ups to scale)
30 Core Twists with feet lifted off ground
40 Standing Calf Raises
50 Jumping Jacks

<u>Workout 2</u>:

3 Rounds For Time:

50 Mountain Climbers
50 Sit-Ups (or abs Workout of Choice)
50 Jumping Jacks
30 Core Twist with feet lifted off ground (Interlock hands)

<u>Workout 3</u>:

3 Rounds For Time:

20 Push-Ups (Knees to Scale)
20 Bench/Chair Dips
50 Side Large Arm Circles Forward
50 Side Large Arm Circles Backwards
50 Front Large Arm Circles (Clockwise)
50 Jumping Jacks

<u>Rest Day</u>

<u>Workout 4:</u>

3- 200 Meter Sprints (No more than 30 Sec Break in
Between Sets)
Then:

3 Rounds For Time:

30 Flutter Kicks
30 Laying Knee to Chest
30 Core Twists with Feet lifted off the ground

<u>Workout 5:</u>

3 Rounds For Time:

20 Air Squats
50 Standing Calf Raises
20 Lunges
50 Jumping Jacks
20 Mountain Climbers

<u>Workout 6:</u>

3 Rounds For Time:

50 Mountain Climbers
20 Push Ups
50 Sit-Ups

<u>Workout 7:</u>

1-10 Pyramid of Push Ups

After each Push Up set:
10 Sit Ups
10 Overhead Air Press

Example of Workout:
1 Push Up
10 Sit Ups
10 Overhead Air Press

2 Push Ups
10 Sit Ups
10 Overhead Air Press

3 Push Ups
10 Sit Ups
10 Overhead Air Press

Continue until reach 10 Push Ups

<u>Rest Day</u>

<u>Workout 8:</u>

3 Rounds For Time:

20 Air Squats
20 1-Leg Chair Split-Squats (10 each Leg)
30 Second Wall Squat (Knees bent 90 Degrees
with back against wall)
50 Sit Ups

<u>Workout 9:</u>

3 Rounds For Time:

20 Incline Push Ups
20 Flutter Kicks
20 Decline Push Ups
20 Flutter Kicks
20 Push Ups
20 Flutter Kicks

<u>Workout 10:</u>

3 Rounds For Time:

25 Air Squats
20 Jumping Lunges
20 Bunny Hops (Calf Raise)
25 Mountain Climbers

<u>Rest Day</u>

<u>Workout 11:</u>

3 Rounds for Time:

200 Meters Run/Jog
25 Push Ups
50 Jumping Jacks
25 Sit Ups

<u>Workout 12:</u>

3 Rounds for Time:

20 Burpees
20 Standing Knee-to-Elbow Cross (Core Exercise)
20 Flutter Kicks

<u>Workout 13:</u>

20-15-10 (Reps per Round)

Push Ups
Sit Ups
Bench Dips
Burpees
Core Twist with Feet Lifted Off the Ground

<u>Workout 14:</u>

1-Mile Run (Timed)

<u>Rest Day</u>

<u>Workout 15:</u>

For Time:

100 Burpees

<u>Workout 16:</u>

3 Rounds for Time:

20 Squats To Jump (Jumping Squats)
20 Standing Calf Raise
20 Jumping Lunges
20 Mountain Climbers

<u>Workout 17:</u>

3 Rounds for Time:

30 Incline Push Ups
30 Sit Ups
30 Overhead Air Press
30 Side Large Arm Circles Forward
30 Side Large Arm Circles Backwards
30 Jumping Jacks

<u>Rest Day</u>

<u>Workout 18:</u>

3 Rounds for Time:

50 High Knees (Bring Knees at least to 90
Degrees while running in place 50 times)
50 Flutter Kicks
50 Knee-To-Elbow Cross (25 Each Side)
50 Jumping Jacks

<u>Workout 19:</u>

For Time:

10- 100 meters run/jog (No more than 30 seconds Rest in Between Sets)

<u>Workout 20:</u>

3 Rounds For Time:

20 Diamond Push Ups (Triceps Push Ups)
20 Side Large Forward Arm Circles
20 Side Large Backwards Arm Circles
20 Bench/Chair Dips
20 Push Ups
20 Flutter Kicks

<u>Rest Day</u>

<u>Workout 21:</u>

3 Rounds for Time:

20 Laying Leg Raises (90 Degree)
20 Incline Push Ups
20 Laying Knees to Chest
20 Decline Push Ups
20 Second Plank (4 Points of Contact activating Core)

<u>Workout 22:</u>

30-20-10

Air Squats
Sit Ups
Lunges
Side to Side Hop (Each Hop is 1 Rep)
Straight Leg Toe Touches

<u>Workout 23:</u>

50 Jumping Jacks
50 Side Small Forward Arm Circles
50 Side Small Backward Arm Circles
50 Overhead Air Press
50 Flutter Kicks

<u>Workout 24:</u>

For Time:

½ Mile As Fast As Possible

<u>Rest Day</u>

<u>Workout 25:</u>

For Time:

100 Jumping Jacks
100 Sit Ups
100 Mountain Climbers
100 Flutter Kicks

<u>Workout 26:</u>

For Time:

100 Push Ups
100 Side Small Forward Arm Circles
100 Side Small Backwards Arm Circles
100 Bench Dips
100 Jumping Jacks

<u>Workout 27:</u>

5 Rounds for Time:

10 Lunges
100 Meters Sprint
10 Air Squats

<u>Workout 28:</u>

3 Rounds for Time:

50 Bunny Hops
50 Side-To-Side Hops
50 Jumping Jacks
50 Core Twists with Feet Lifted

<u>Rest Day</u>

<u>Workout 29:</u>

3 Rounds for Time:

30 Seconds Wall Sit (Legs 90 degrees back
against wall)
30 Second Plank
30 Second Left Side Plank
30 Second Right Side Plank
30 Air Squats
30 Standing Calf Raise

<u>Workout 30:</u>

3 Rounds for Time:

20 Burpees
20 Push Ups
50 Bunny Hops
20 Bench Dips
50 Jumping Jacks

<u>Workout 31:</u>

3 Rounds for Time:

25 Jumping Squats
30 Jumping Lunges
35 Standing Calf Raise
40 Jumping Jacks
45 Crunches (Sit Up Substitution)

<u>Workout 32:</u>

For Time:

Jog/Run 1.5 Miles

<u>Rest Day</u>

<u>Workout 33:</u>

3 Rounds for Time:

50 Standing Twists
50 Flutter Kicks
50 Jumping Jacks
50 Mountain Climbers

<u>Workout 34:</u>

3 Rounds for Time:

30 Squat Jumps (Jump Squats)
20 Jumping Lunges
30 Bunny Hops
20 Standing Knees-to-Elbow Crossover
20 Jumping Jacks

<u>Workout 35:</u>

3 Rounds for Time:

20 Incline Push Ups
20 Bench Dips
50 Jumping Jacks
20 Decline Push Ups
20 Diamond Push Ups

<u>Rest Day</u>

<u>Workout 36:</u>

For Time:

10 – 100 Meters Sprints (No More than 20 Seconds Rest In Between Sprints)

<u>Workout 37:</u>

3 Rounds for Time:

25 Left Leg Chair/Bench Step Ups
25 Right Leg Chair/Bench Step Ups
25 Air Squats
20 Back Leg Lunges
25 Bunny Hops

<u>Workout 38:</u>

3 Rounds for Time:

25 Push Ups
25 Side Small Forward Arm Circles
25 Side Small Backwards Arm Circles
25 Front Arm Circles (Clockwise)
25 Decline Push Ups
25 Crunches (Substitute with Sit Ups)

<u>Rest Day</u>

<u>Workout 39:</u>

For Time:

Run/Jog 1 Mile

<u>Workout 40:</u>

3 Rounds for Time:

20 Squats
25 Left Side Crunches
25 Right Side Crunches
20 Standing Calf Raises
40 Lunges

Workout 41:

10 Rounds for Time:

10 Push Ups
20 Sit Ups
10 Bench Dips

Workout 42:

3 Rounds for Time:

20 Lunges
30 Calf Raise
20 Air Squats
30 Crunches (Sit Ups Substitution)
200 Meters Run

Rest Day

Workout 43:

3 Rounds for Time:

20 Lunges
250 Meters Sprint
20 Air Squats
20 Standing Calf Raise

<u>Workout 44:</u>

3 Rounds for Time:

20 Sit Ups
20 Core Twist with feet Lifted off ground
20 Flutter Kicks
20 Laying Knees to Chest
20 Mountain Climbers

<u>Workout 45:</u>

3 Rounds for Time:

20 Incline Push Ups
50 Jumping Jacks
20 Decline Push Ups
50 Jumping Jacks
20 Push Ups
50 Jumping Jacks

<u>Workout 46:</u>

For Time:

Run/Walk 2 Miles

<u>Rest Day</u>

<u>Workout 47:</u>

5 Rounds for Time:

20 Push Ups
20 Bench Dips
40 Crunches (Sit Ups for Substitution)

<u>Workout 48:</u>

For Time:

50 Lunges (25 Each Leg)
5-Minute Jog/Run
50 Air Squats
50 Standing Calf Raise

<u>Workout 49:</u>

3 Rounds for Time:

20 Burpees
20 Push Ups
20 Bench/Chair Dips
50 Crunches (Sit Up Substitution)

<u>Rest Day</u>

<u>Workout 50:</u>

10 Rounds for Time:

10 Air Squats
100 Meters Run/Jog
20 Standing Calf Raise

<u>Workout 51:</u>

For Time:

50 Mountain Climbers
50 Push Ups
50 Bench Dips
50 Jumping Jacks
50 Sit Ups

<u>Workout 52:</u>

3 Rounds for Time:

25 Air Squat Jumps (Jumping Air Squats)
50 Sit Ups
20 Jumping Lunges
50 Standing Calf Raise
50 Core Twist with feet lifted off the ground

<u>Workout 53:</u>

3 Rounds for Time:

50 Standing Knees-to-Elbow Cross (25 Each
Side)
50 Side Small Forward Arm Circles
50 Side Small Backwards Arm Circles
25 Push Ups
25 Bench Dips
50 Flutter Kicks

<u>Rest Day</u>

<u>Workout 54:</u>

3 Rounds for Time:

25 Diamond Push Ups
50 Jumping Jacks
25 Bench/Chair Dips
50 Jumping Jacks
25 Push Ups

<u>Workout 55:</u>

3 Rounds for Time:

10 Burpees
15 Air Squats
20 Lunges (10 Each Leg)
25 Mountain Climbers
50 Sit Ups (Crunches Substitution)

<u>Workout 56:</u>

3 Rounds for Time:

50 Jumping Jacks
50 Bunny Hops
50 Side-to-Side Hops
50 Flutter Kicks

<u>Workout 57:</u>

3 Rounds for Time:

500 Meters Run/Jog (No more than 30 seconds
rest in between rounds)

<u>Rest Day</u>

<u>Workout 58:</u>

3 Rounds for Time:

50 Flutter Kicks
50 Crunches (Sit Ups Substitution)
50 Jumping Jacks
50 Bunny Hops
50 Lunges (25 Each Leg)

<u>Workout 59:</u>

5 Rounds for Time:

20 Air Squats
200 Meters Run
20 Push Ups

<u>Workout 60:</u>

For Time:

1-Mile Jog (Throughout Jog Sprint 10 Seconds at
Least 10 Times)

<u>Workout 61:</u>

3 Rounds for Time:

15 Burpees
20 Push Ups
25 Bench/Chair Dips
30 Flutter Kicks
35 Mountain Climbers
40 Sit Ups (Crunches Substitution)

<u>Rest Day</u>

<u>Workout 62:</u>

3 Rounds for Time:

45 Second Wall Sit
45 Second Plank
45 Second Left Side Plank
45 Second Right Side Plank
45 Air Squats

<u>Workout 63:</u>

3 Rounds for Time:

20 Burpees
30 Push Ups
30 Bench Dips
30 Incline Push Ups
30 Diamond Push Ups

<u>Workout 64:</u>

5 Rounds for Time:

20 Air Squats
20 Lunges (10 Each Leg)
20 Mountain Climbers
20 Flutter Kicks
20 Core Twists with feet lifted (Russian Twists)

<u>Workout 65:</u>

5 Rounds for Time:

250 Meter Sprint (No more than 15 second rest
in between rounds)

<u>Rest Day</u>

Workout 66:

3 Rounds for Time:

30 Push Ups
30 Bench Dips
30 Side Small Forward Arm Circles
30 Side Small Backward Arm Circles
30 Air Overhead Press
30 Flutter Kicks
30 Mountain Climbers

Workout 67:

3 Rounds for Time:

30 Split Squats (15 Each Leg)
30 Standing Straight Leg Toe Touches
30 Laying Knee-to-Chest (Substitution Crunches)
30 Squat Jumps (Jump Squats)
30 Jumping Jacks

Workout 68:

5 Rounds for Time:

15 Burpees
30 Mountain Climbers
15 Push Ups
30 Jumping Jacks

<u>Workout 69:</u>

3 Rounds for Time:

25 Bench Dips
25 Crunches (Substitution Sit Ups)
25 Diamond Push Ups
25 Flutter Kicks
25 Mountain Climbers

<u>Rest Day</u>

<u>Workout 70:</u>

5 Rounds for Time:

10 Burpees
100 Meters Sprint
20 Crunches (Substitution Sit Ups)

<u>Workout 71:</u>

3 Rounds for Time:

50 Bench/Chair Step Ups (25 Each Leg)
30 Jumping Squats
50 Bunny Hops
30 Jumping Lunges
50 Crunches (Substitution Sit Ups)

<u>Workout 72:</u>

3 Rounds for Time:

20 Push Ups
20 Bench Dips
20 Incline Push Ups
20 Bench Dips
20 Decline Push Ups
20 Bench Dips

<u>Rest Day</u>

<u>Workout 73:</u>

For Time:

100 Jumping Jacks
100 Sit Ups
100 Mountain Climbers
100 Flutter Kicks
1000 Meters Jog/Run

<u>Workout 74:</u>

5 Rounds for Time:

25 Air Squats
200 Meters Sprint
20 Lunges

Workout 75:

5 Rounds for Time:

15 Mountain Climbers
15 Push Ups
15 Bench Dips
15 Burpees

Workout 76:

For Time:

Jog/Run 1 Mile
50 Air Squats
Jog/Run 1 Mile

Rest Day

Workout 77:

3 Rounds for Time:

50 Standing Knees-to-Elbows Cross
50 Jumping Jacks
50 Flutter Kicks
50 Side-to-Side Hops
50 Mountain Climbers

<u>Workout 78:</u>

5 Rounds for Time:

25 Air Squat Jumps (Jump Squats)
250 Meters Jog/Run
30 Jumping Lunges
25 Flutter Kicks

<u>Workout 79:</u>

3 Rounds for Time:

25 Push Ups
25 Bench/Chair Dips
25 Incline Push Ups
25 Flutter Kicks
25 Decline Push Ups
25 Crunches (Substitution Sit Ups)

<u>Workout 80:</u>

30-20-10

Air Squats
Crunches (Substitution Sit Ups)
Lunges (Each Leg)
Standing Calf Raise
Mountain Climbers

<u>Rest Day</u>

<u>Workout 81:</u>

3 Rounds for Time:

20 Meters Bear Crawl
50 Mountain Climbers
20 Burpees
50 Jumping Jacks

<u>Workout 82:</u>

3 Rounds for Time:

30 Bench Dips
30 Front Small Arm Circles (Clockwise)
30 Side Forward Small Arm Circles
30 Side Backward Arm Circles
30 Overhead Air Press
30 Push Ups
30 Flutter Kicks

<u>Workout 83:</u>

5 Rounds for Time:

25 Air Squats
250 Meters Jog/Run
20 Burpees
20 Lunges (10 Each Leg)

<u>Workout 84:</u>

3 Rounds for Time:

50 Push Ups
50 Flutter Kicks
50 Bench Dips
50 Jumping Jacks
50 Mountain Climbers

<u>Rest Day</u>

<u>Workout 85:</u>

For Time:

2-Mile Jog

<u>Workout 86:</u>

Max Repetitions (1 Minute Break Between
Workouts):

2 Minutes of Flutter Kicks
2 Minutes of Jumping Jacks
2 Minutes of Push Ups
2 Minutes of Sit Ups
2 Minutes of Mountain Climbers

<u>Workout 87:</u>

As Many Rounds as Possible in 15 Minutes:

20 Lunges (10 Each Leg)
20 Bench Dips
20 Air Squats
20 Crunches/Sit Ups

<u>Workout 88:</u>

5 Rounds for Time:

10 Incline Push Ups
10 Sit Ups
10 Decline Push Ups
10 Sit Ups
10 Push Ups
10 Sit Ups
100 Jumping Jacks

<u>Rest Day</u>

<u>Workout 89:</u>

3 Rounds for Time:

15 Burpees
25 Jumping Squats
30 Jumping Lunges
35 Standing Calf Raise
40 Bunny Hops
50 Side-to-Side Hops

<u>Workout 90:</u>

3 Rounds for Time:

30 Push Ups
30 Flutter Kicks
30 Bench Dips
30 Core Twists with Feet Lifted
30 Side Large Forward Arm Circles
30 Side Large Backward Arm Circles
30 Mountain Climbers
30 Front Arm Circles (Counter-Clockwise)

<u>Workout 91:</u>

3 Rounds for Time:

50 Air Squats
500 Meters Jog/Run
50 Bunny Hops

<u>Workout 92:</u>

3 Rounds for Time:

50 Core Twists with Feet Lifted
50 Flutter Kicks
50 Bench Dips
50 Incline Push Ups
50 Mountain Climbers

<u>Rest Day</u>

<u>Workout 93:</u>

10 Rounds for Time:

Sprint for 30 Seconds
20 Push Ups

<u>Workout 94:</u>

3 Rounds for Repetitions:

30 Seconds of Plank
30 Seconds of Mountain Climbers
30 Seconds of Left Side Plank
30 Seconds of Jumping Jacks
30 Seconds of Right Side Plank
30 Seconds of Sit Ups
30 Seconds of Core Twists with Feet Lifted

<u>Workout 95:</u>

3 Rounds for Time:

50 Jumping Air Squats
25 Burpees
50 Jumping Lunges
25 Bunny Hops
50 Side-to-Side Hops

Workout 96:

3 Rounds for Time:

50 Push Ups
25 Flutter Kicks
50 Mountain Climbers
25 Overhead Air Press
50 Front Small Arm Circles (Clockwise)
25 Sit Ups

Rest Day

Workout 97:

2 Rounds for Time:

1-Mile Jog/Run
50 Standing Knee-To-Elbow Cross (25 Each Side)
50 Jumping Jacks
50 Flutter Kicks

Workout 98:

3 Rounds for Time:

25 Push Ups
25 Bench Dips
25 Decline Push Ups
25 Burpees
25 Incline Push Ups
25 Mountain Climbers
25 Sit Ups

<u>Workout 99:</u>

For Time:

99 Flutter Kicks
99 Jumping Jacks
99 Mountain Climbers
99 Core Twists with Feet Lifted
99 Bunny Hops

<u>Workout 100:</u>

For Time:

100 Push Ups
100 Air Squats
100 Flutter Kicks
100 Bench Dips
100 Burpees

Enjoy the rest of your new fitness journey! Be on the look out for more books covering fitness and other motivational/life-changing material. Thanks for working out with me!

Next are some of the exercises explained to the best of my ability based off training, experience, and second hand knowledge.

I will attempt to explain the exercises used in this program but it is often quicker to complete a simple search on the Internet for a demonstration video of the exercise. All of the exercises used in this program are common and there is plenty of information about how to properly perform each movement on the internet. Videos and pictures often help explain exercises when words cannot.
DO NOT attempt to do an exercise you do not understand because the risk of injury. Ensure you have a complete understanding and concept of the workout and the proper way to conduct the movement before you begin.

Good luck on your fitness journey and I hope I was able to help by publishing The Ultimate No Equipment Fitness Program.

<u>Exercise Descriptions:</u>

Push Ups-
Lay flat on the ground with your belly pressed against the floor. Place your hands shoulder width apart in line with your nipples. Keep your legs close together or touching. From that position, facing forward, push up but straightening arms. Do not Arch back; keep back in a straight line.

Decline Push Ups-
Place your feet in an elevated position. (Example-chair, bench, couch, bed) With feet elevated and chest on floor. Place hands shoulder width apart in line with your nipples. Keep your legs close together or touching. With your head forward, push straight up by straightening your arms. Repeat as necessary to complete repetitions required by workout. Do not arch back or allow curve in spine; keep back in a straight line.

Incline Push Ups-
Place your hands in an elevated position. (Example-chair, bench, couch, bed) Position your hands shoulder width apart in line with your nipples. Keep your legs close together or touching. With your head forward, push straight up by straightening your arms. Do not arch back or allow curve in spine, keep back in straight line.

Diamond Push Ups-
Laying flat on the ground, place your hands under your chest approximately 2 inches apart creating a "diamond" shape with your hands. With your legs spread apart for adequate balance, push up by straightening arms. Do not arch back or allow curve in spine. Keep back in straight line.

Bench Dips-
Sitting on the bench/chair, position your hands next to your bottom, shoulder width apart. From this position, extend your legs and drop your bottom off the bench or chair. Holding yourself up with your arms, bend elbows to allow body to lower towards ground. Bring elbows down to form a 90-degree angle.

Squats-
With your feet shoulder width apart, drop your butt back towards the back of your heels pretending to sit back on the toilet or an imaginary chair. Keep your knees over your ankles the entire time while keeping your feet firmly planted on the ground. Do not allow your knees to move over your feet or your butt to drop directly to your feet. Drop your butt down until your knees and legs form a 90* or greater angle and then explode back up keeping your feet planted.

Jump Squats / Squat Jumps –
Preform the same exercise as above but when you explode back up from the squat position, jump as high as possible in the air.

Bunny Hops-
With your feet together, jump up and down keeping the landing and jump on the ball of your feet. This motion will be the same as if one were to jump over a jump rope. Each time the feet come off the ground, into the air, and back down to the ground counts as one repetition.

Side-to-Side Hops-
With your feet together, visually find or make a line on the ground. Focusing on that line, hop from one side of the line to the other. The jump will be approximately 2-6 inches off the ground. Each times your feet land on one side of the line, it counts as one repetition.

Lunges-
Starting position will be standing, feet together. From this position, take a large stride forward. Once the foot is forward, drop both knees towards the ground. Your front leg/thigh will should be parallel with the ground when lowered properly. From this position (lowered), lift yourself from the ground upward while keeping your feet planted in the same position. Once up bring your front leg back and repeat with the other leg. If this exercise is hard on your knees then only go down ½ way or substitute for a different leg exercise.

Jumping Lunges-
This workout will be the same as the lunges but when one of your legs is forward, from the downward parallel position, explode, jumping into the air and moving your back leg to the front and front leg to the back. Land on the ground with approximately the same leg spacing you previously had and immediately drop to a lunge. Once landed, the previous back leg will now be the front leg and parallel thigh.

Sit Ups-
Lie on the ground with your knees slightly bent (approximately 45* angle) and arms in a crossed position across the chest. From this position, raise the upper body off the ground reaching your elbows to your knees. Once your elbows touch your knees then go back down to the ground to complete 1 repetition.

Flutter Kicks-
Laying flat on the ground, place your hands under your hips to help relieve lower back strain. From this position, lift both legs, together and touching, 6 inches off the ground. Keep legs 6 inches off the ground for the entire exercise, never touching the ground. From 6 inches off the ground, raise one leg approximately 24-36 inches keeping the other straight and 6 inches off the ground. As this leg comes down raise the other leg 24-36 inches changing the high and low leg. 1 repetition is completed when both legs have been in the UP position.

Core Twists with Feet Lifted-
From the Sit Up Position, lift your feet a couple inches off the ground. With your hands joined together in front of your stomach and your feet lifted, move your hands from one hip to the other. Each time, touch your hands (together) on the ground beside your left then right side. Each time you touch the ground counts as one repetition.

Front Small Arm Circles-
Standing with feet shoulder width apart, extend your arms straight out in front of your body with palms facing towards the ground. You arms should be directly in line with your shoulder creating a 90 Degree angle with your body. From here move your arms in small circles either clockwise or counterclockwise depending on the workout.

Side Small/Large Arm Circles-
Standing with feet shoulder width apart, extend your arms out to the side of your body keeping your palms facing the ground. From here conduct either large or small arm circles, backwards and forwards.

Standing Knee-to-Elbow Cross-
Standing with feet shoulder width a part place your hands behind your head with your elbows extended past your head. Take your Left elbow and crunch your body down bringing it towards your right knee. At the same time, bring your right knee up towards your stomach meeting your elbow right at your belly button. Bring your body back to the starting position and repeat with the Right Elbow and Left Knee.

Mountain Climbers-
From the Push Up Position bring one knee (leg) up to your chest in a running position. From this position you will bring the back leg forward and the forward leg back. Each time the legs cross and land counts as one repetition. For demonstration video search online for "Mountain Climbers Exercise Video Demonstration".

Plank-
Lying on the ground, lift your body off the ground like the push up but with your forearms. In other words, make your arms/elbow a 90-degree angle with your elbows aligned under your shoulders. With the forearms resting on the ground, hold your body off the ground like a push up in the up position resting on your forearms. Hold this position, flexing your core and squeezing your gluteus (butt). This position will be held for the allotted time in workout.

Side Plank-
The side plank is performed like the regular plank but from either the left or right side. Lying on one side, align your elbow under your shoulder and lift your body off the ground. With just the forearm and one foot touching the ground while the other foot rests on top, hold your body in the lifted position for the allotted time in the workout. This can be preformed on either the left or right side of the body. For more clarification and information on the workout search, "Plank and Side Plank Exercise Videos".

Burpees-
From a Standing Position, drop your butt down like a squat and on your way down, thrust your legs back and drop down into the "down" push up position. Once your Chest hits the ground, push up. Thrust your legs back to bring your body to the down squat position. From here, thrust up and jump in the air. This exercise is fairly complex and searching for a video will help clarify the movements if one is not familiar with a burpee.

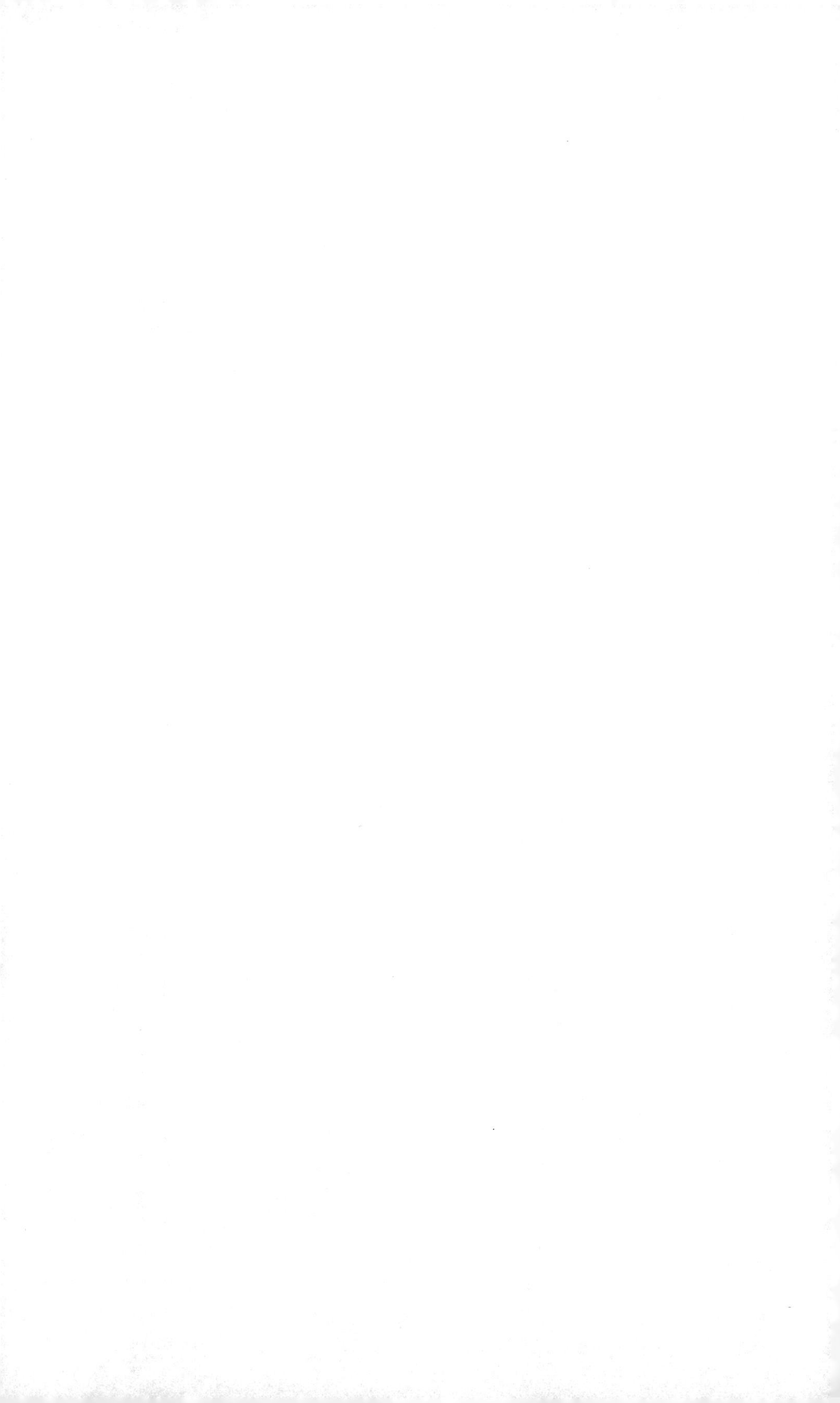